My Jonah Journey

DEVELOPING AN
ATTITUDE OF GRATITUDE

Linda M. Brandt

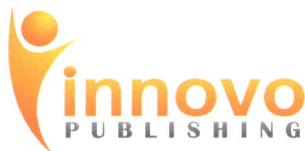

innovo
PUBLISHING

Published by
Innovo Publishing LLC
www.innovopublishing.com
1-888-546-2111

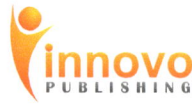

Providing Full-Service Publishing Services for
Christian Authors, Artists, and Organizations: Hardbacks, Paperbacks,
eBooks, Audiobooks, Music, and Film

MY JONAH JOURNEY:
DEVELOPING AN ATTITUDE OF GRATITUDE

ISBN 13: 978-1-61314-145-8

Cover Design & Interior Layout by Innovo Publishing LLC
Cover Art & Illustrations by Linda M. Brandt

Printed in the United States of America
U.S. Printing History
First Edition: April 2013

PREFACE

In 2002, my son, Scott, was killed by a drunk driver. He was only thirty-two. Scottie was tall, handsome, creative, and funny. He was the father of a little girl and boy and had another baby boy due any day. His life was snuffed out in seconds, and to this day I can barely speak of it. It feels like a permanent kick to my stomach.

Two years after the death of my son, I was diagnosed with an extremely rare and serious brain tumor. I had always wanted so much out of life—success, creative expression, recognition. Now any hope to ever attain these things was gone. I was overcome with despair and in desperate need of a savior.

I titled my autobiography *My Jonah Journey* because Jonah's story, like mine, is not so much about being swallowed as it is about being separated from God and confronting the storms of life. While living "inside the belly of the whale," God revealed Himself to Jonah—and to me—as a loving, caring, creative Presence who is willing and able to transform the terror of the storm into a peaceful calm.

I pray that with the Holy Spirit's blessing, reading my story will change your life—that you will find courage, inspiration, and comfort. The storms in our lives can bring heavy bumps and bruises, but know this, my friend—the Captain of your soul can be trusted. Put your trust in Him today.

—Linda M. Brandt

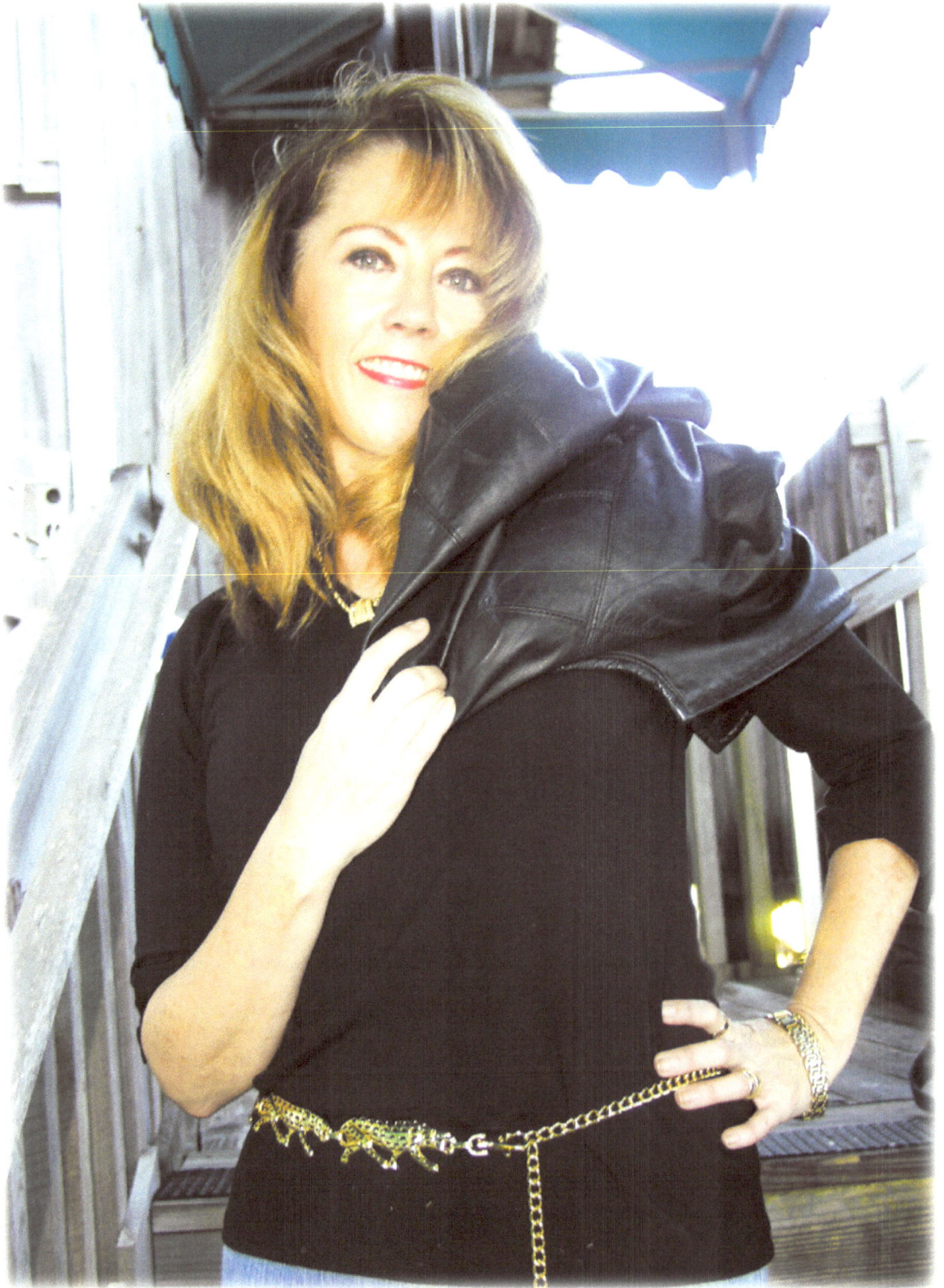

Author-Artist, Linda M. Brandt

MY JONAH JOURNEY

If I just do this one thing, if I just get this one thing, if I just meet this one person, my life will be perfect. Have these ever been your thoughts? If so, then like I was, you are a person who dreams of escaping reality, who longs for the intangible, invincible, and most likely, the impossible. Hey, who hasn't had thoughts like these at one time or another? Even Jonah, a prophet of the Lord, once tried to dodge the life God had planned for him.

Now the word of the LORD came to Jonah the son of Amittai, saying, ² "Arise, go to Nineveh, that great city, and cry out against it; for their wickedness has come up before Me." ³ But Jonah arose to flee to Tarshish from the presence of the LORD. He went down to Joppa, and found a ship going to Tarshish; so he paid the fare, and went down into it, to go with them to Tarshish from the presence of the LORD.

⁴ But the LORD sent out a great wind on the sea, and there was a mighty tempest on the sea, so that the ship was about to be broken up. ⁵ Then the mariners were afraid; and every man cried out to his god, and threw the cargo that *was* in the ship into the sea, to lighten the load. But Jonah had gone down into the lowest parts of the ship, had lain down, and was fast asleep. ⁶ So the captain came to him, and said to him, "What do you mean, sleeper? Arise, call on your God; perhaps your God will consider us, so that we may not perish." ⁷ And they said to one another, "Come, let us cast lots, that we may know for whose cause this trouble *has come* upon us." So they cast lots, and the lot fell on Jonah. ⁸ Then they said to him, "Please tell us! For whose cause *is* this trouble upon us? What is your occupation? And where do you come from? What is your country? And of what people are you?" ⁹ So he said to them, "I *am* a Hebrew; and I fear the LORD, the God of heaven, who made the sea and the dry *land.*" ¹⁰ Then the men were exceedingly afraid, and said to him, "Why have you done this?" For the men knew that he fled from the presence of the LORD, because he had told them. ¹¹ Then they said to him, "What shall we do to you that the sea may be calm for us?"—for the sea was growing more tempestuous. ¹² And he said to them, "Pick me up and throw me into the sea; then the sea will become calm for you. For I know that this great tempest *is* because of me" (Jonah 1:1-12).

Everyone on that boat, including Jonah, was convinced that if Jonah was thrown into the sea, life would be calm and peaceful again. So they threw him overboard and returned to their fish nets and to the daily grind of living on a boat. And indeed it *was* more peaceful—for a time.

But what about Jonah? Well, Jonah was now lying in the belly of a whale, where all he could do was contemplate—and contemplate he did.[1] It must have been pretty scary for him in those dark and torrential waves—not to mention the fierceness and blackness of that monstrous whale mouth swallowing him up.

I was very much like Jonah and his shipmates until April 9 of 2004. I had my life pretty well planned out, and anything not directly helping me attain my goals and dreams was "thrown overboard." By God's grace, I was blessed with a beautiful, loving family and boatloads of wonderful friends. I had exotic island homes, traveled extensively, ate in the finest restaurants, drank the finest wines, and had access to lots of important people.

Even though I had lost my beautiful firstborn child, Scottie, just two years earlier in a horrible automobile accident, I had continued to trust God and believe that He wouldn't have taken my beautiful "little boy" without good reason. I could not have imagined the most unusual way in which God would bring Scottie back into my life.

It was Good Friday and a beautiful sunny day in St. Augustine, Florida. I had been commuting from my art studio in the Gulf of Mexico to this beautiful Atlantic location where I painted sometimes twenty-four hours without stopping, except for an occasional nap and bite to eat. On this particular Friday, Jimmy, my husband at the time, and I had decided to eat lunch on the beach before loading up our cars and heading west to conduct weekend business at our restaurant in Cedar Key.

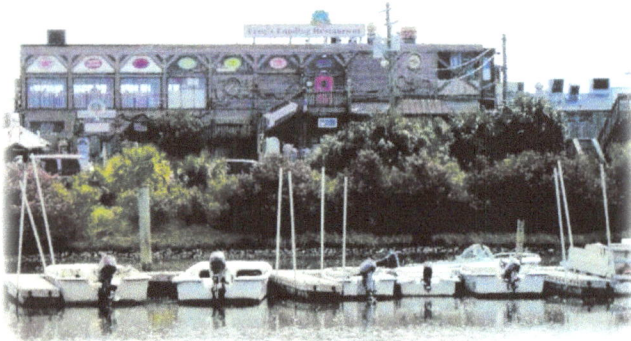

Frog's Landing, our restaurant in Cedar Key

The sun was quite warm as we sat outside sipping ice cold drinks and reading the newspaper. I suddenly felt unusually hot and asked if we could sit inside. We moved inside to a cooler location, but I continued to feel faint and confused. I asked where the restroom was

---

[1] Now the LORD had prepared a great fish to swallow Jonah. And Jonah was in the belly of the fish three days and three nights. (Jonah 1:17)

so I could get my head down. Our waitress set our salads on the counter, and as I stood to try to get to the restroom, l looked at my husband and said, "This isn't working." It was then that I felt concrete smashing under my right temple and blood oozing from my head. Everything went black.

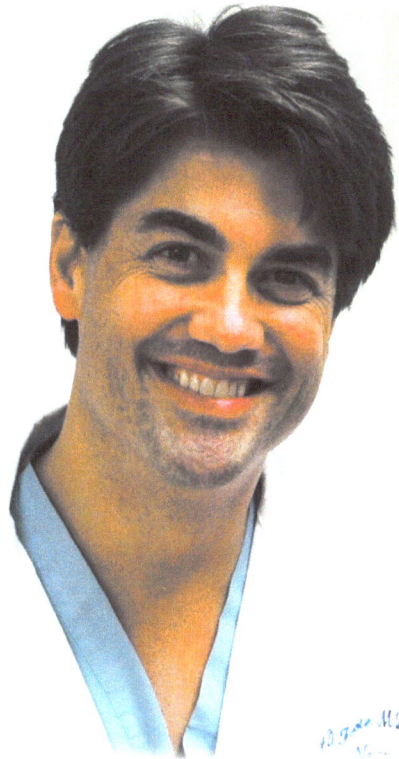

Dr. Kelly Foote, my neurosurgeon

The lights were red and flashing and the sirens screaming as the ambulance hurried me to the local hospital. I came to in the emergency room. A young man who had tended to me in the ambulance introduced himself as Craig and told me he was putting me in the hands of the ER doctor but asked if he could pray for me before releasing me to him. I said of course, and right there in the ambulance, he knelt down beside the gurney, took my hand, and prayed a sweet little prayer asking God to watch over me and help me through this time. My Jonah journey had begun, and God was with me. Perhaps you are wondering if God is with you in your journey. He is, my friend, He is—even in the darkest, scariest times of your life.

Towards evening—at least the light through my hospital window resembled early evening—I saw a doctor holding up film to the window and Jimmy standing beside him looking at it. The doctor spoke softly. They shook their heads and then walked slowly to my bedside.

The doctor began with, "What you have is very, very serious. You have a large tumor at the base of your brain. It is a very delicate operation, and we are transporting you to another hospital for the surgery." I pushed back the tears then once again drifted into unconsciousness.

My husband and I had cancelled our hospital insurance several months earlier because it had become extremely expensive. We were non-smokers, fit, and healthy (or so we thought). Besides, we had twenty-five employees to whom we needed to pay salaries and benefits. We had been looking for an alternative insurance company for ourselves but without luck.

Three days later, somewhat hazy but conscious, there were the lights and ambulance noises again. I was thankful to be getting help at the "new" hospital—especially since I had no insurance. The men in the ambulance brought me through the emergency room, up the elevators, and into a hall where I was taken to the neurosurgery ward. What I remember most was seeing all the shaven heads, empty stares, and lots of tubes. The sights and smells nauseated me, and I began to fear for my life.

I'm not sure when the "new" doctor appeared, but I believe it was late that afternoon. He looked more like a rock star than a brain surgeon. He was in his thirties, with dark, thick, disheveled hair, and a smile as brilliant and beautiful as I had ever seen. *Wow!* I thought to myself. *I guess I'll be okay. At least I have someone magnificent to look at!*

That magnificent someone was Dr. Kelly Foote, who was explaining to me that although my procedure had originally been planned for early the next morning, after conferring with the other neurosurgeons, he believed he must take action and "go in" immediately. He said that tentacles from the tumor had lodged around the fourth ventricle of my brain stem, and it had swollen and backed up. Should the brain stem erupt, which could happen at any moment, they would have thirty minutes to save my life, which would not give them enough time even to open up the cranial bone. Remembering those empty stares, I reluctantly asked Dr. Foote what the consequences of this surgery could possibly mean to my quality of life. Dr. Foote humbly confessed, "There could be death, disability, we just don't know."

I said, "I have two requests; first, I must continue to paint!" Dr. Foote was quick to point out that that was entirely up to God. I thought to myself, *Surely God will keep me painting. It has been my passion for my whole life. And after all, He showed up in my art all the time!* I found peace in these thoughts. "Okay, this is my second request: No skateboarder hairdos." I had seen all those half-shaven heads, and I did not want one! The doctor smiled a beautiful smile and said, "That I can work with." But somehow I had the feeling my journey was not going to be about hairdos. I was about to enter the "belly of the whale!"

The next morning, they came and got me. My beautiful daughter, Christie, had been staying with me at the hospital. My big, strapping, handsome son, Mike, was in Ohio. I wanted to put my arms around them both and hold them tight. I knew this might be the last time I saw them. I was lifted onto a gurney and taken down some halls and into the operating room. There I lay on my back drifting in and out of a sleepy state. Had there been something in my IV to make me so tired, or was my brain in a state of numbness? Was this really happening, or was I just dreaming?

The surgeons all entered in mask and gown (there seemed to be quite a few of them), and there was Dr. Foote. A young female stood next to him. Her eyes looked familiar; I think she had been in my room earlier.

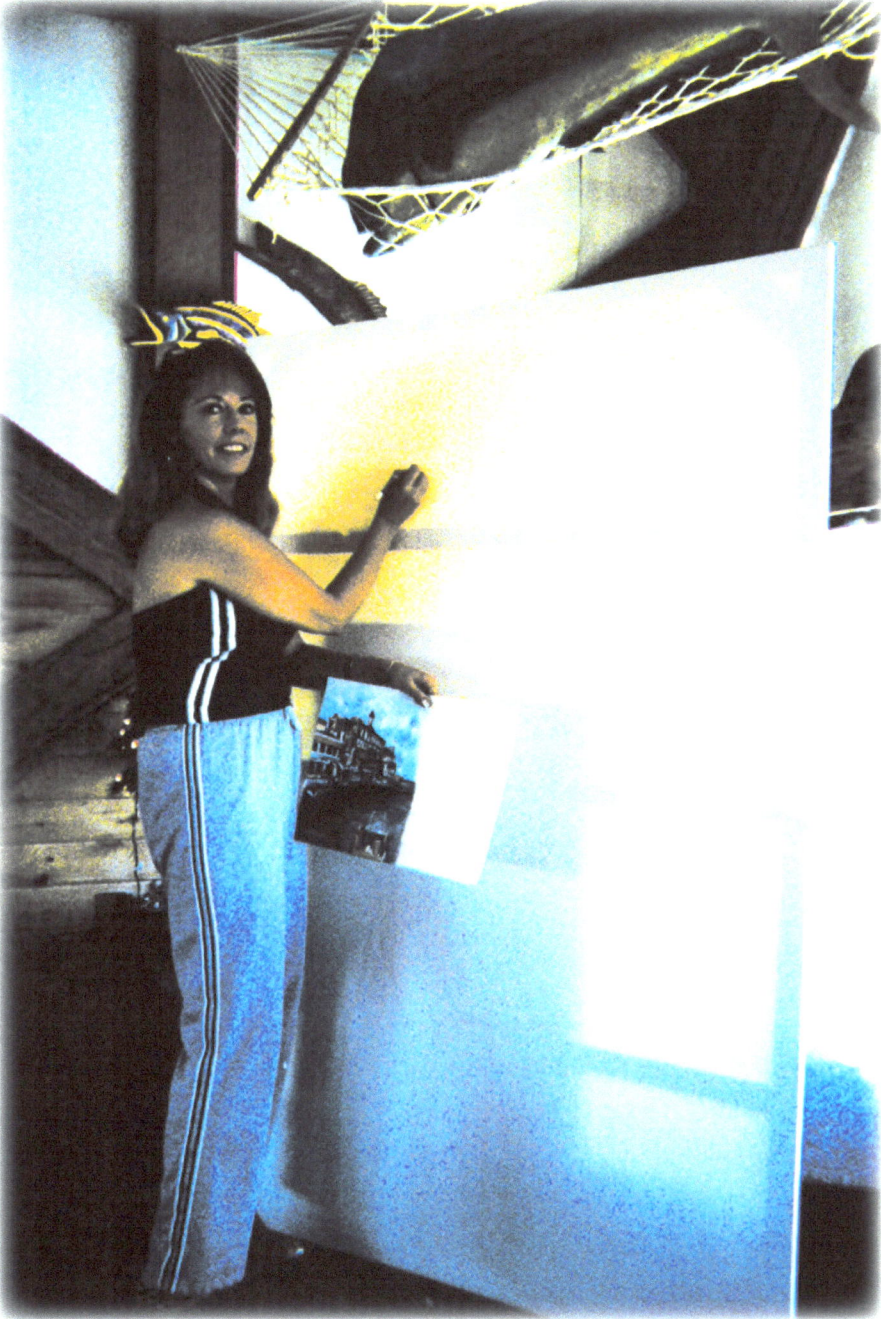

Me at the canvas, doing what I love most

Then I heard very soft footsteps behind my head—almost undetectable. I felt a hand on my shoulder. I looked around, expecting to lock eyes with my attentive anesthesiologist. But what was this? How could it be? It was Scottie, my Scottie! He said, "I'm here, Mom. Everything's going to be all right." Peace invaded my being from head to toe. I looked at that young, handsome doctor and asked, "We going to be okay?" He bumped shoulders with the young female doctor next to him and gave me a thumbs-up. Yes, I was going to be okay—somehow. I don't remember anything that happened after that until I awoke in the recovery room.

My family tells me it was a nearly ten-and-a-half-hour surgery. Dr. Foote kept them informed when he could. Out in the waiting room, some of my family, friends, and clergy had come to pray for me. Prayer surrounded me and upheld me.

MIDLINE SUBOCCIPITAL CRANIOTOMY, C1 LAMINECTOMY, TELO-VELO-TONSILAR AND TRANSVERMIAN APPROACH TO RESECTION OF A CEREBELLAR AND FOURTH VENTRICULAR MASS.

RIGHT FRONTAL VENTRICULOSTOMY FOR TREATMENT OF OBSTRUCTIVE HYDROCEPHALUS

Doctor's orders for my brain surgery

The brain is a funny thing, especially after being exposed to air. It's the central core of your being, and it does not like to be exposed. When it is, it feels threatened—very, very threatened.

I awoke in recovery. *My daughter…where is she?* I panicked. I felt sick—so very sick. Warm liquid was oozing out of my eyes and ears. I felt like I was dying. *My daughter, Christie… Where is she?* The room was spinning. *She is trying to protect me, and they want to hurt her!* Christie's husband, John, a deputy sheriff, was there. *They are trying to kill me, and they want the whole thing over before going off their shift!*

Christie reached for John's gun. They shot her! *My God, they have killed her!* John was begging them to help her and to help me. The room was still spinning. I was grabbing the doctor's arms. I wanted to remember their descriptions.

As an artist, police sketches had been my specialty. *I'll get their descriptions, and I'll get justice.* Flashing lights like cameras were going off. They were taking my picture. *Why are they taking my picture? They want evidence of my death! They're putting a sheet over my head, but I won't die. I feel my life blood oozing from me, but I will not die!*

One man, in particular, was taking care of me. *I will get his bone description. His eyes are blue.* I didn't feel human. I didn't feel alive. *Where am I? What is happening?* I heard a woman talking to the man, who was whistling softly while he was working on me. *This feels like an Alfred Hitchcock movie. He must be an undertaker.* She whispered, "She heard." *They now know that I am on to them. He is hurrying. His shift is almost over. They want me dead and prepared for cremation before he leaves. No evidence.*

The next morning, new doctors entered the recovery room. An attractive, blonde, female doctor was holding my chart. I remembered her. Her name was Pam, and I had met her the day the doctors surrounded my bed before surgery. Was that just two days ago? She and a male doctor with glasses were shouting corrective orders to the recovery room staff. She was saving my life. *Thank God, I have hung on! I'll be okay now. My daughter, though… where is my beautiful daughter?* I drifted again into unconsciousness.

Later I awoke in a regular room. The back of my head was stapled, and there was a drain tube out the front of my head. The right side of my head was scabbed from the fall. I had my hair but, unfortunately, it was not too pretty. Days later, my daughter and mother-in-law tried to dry wash it. My husband's parents were by my bedside. My father-in-law fed me orange sorbet. Amazingly, it tasted really wonderful.

My mother called, but I couldn't stand the sound of the phone up to my ear. The noise was excruciating. I wanted to see her, I wanted to talk to her, but light and sound nauseated me. My mother-in-law gently and wisely touched my arm and said, "Honey, it's your mother. Please talk to her just for a moment. She needs to hear your voice." She laid the phone on my pillow, away from my ear.

Mom tearfully expressed her and Dad's love and prayers for me. I so wanted them to be there with me, and I should have asked them to come. It's just that I was determined to get well and go home, and I knew I'd need them to be there with me even more then. A mom and dad's love surpasses everything.

People sometimes ask me if I ever noticed anything different about myself before I blacked out that day at the seaside restaurant. And, yes, you could say that I had symptoms, except at the time I didn't know they were symptoms.

I had been burning the candle at both ends and thought I was just really tired. Then there was the time I fell off of my bike—twice, actually—and both times, on my left shoulder. Walking had become difficult, too. I had the tendency to fall to my left.

Six weeks before the beach incident, I awoke with a start at one o'clock in the morning. My head was on fire, my insides were on fire, and I had excruciating pain running down my left arm. Fearing I was having a heart attack, I got up and took four aspirin and four ibuprofen. An hour later, the pain had not dissipated, so I again took the same dose.

After about twenty minutes, I fell asleep. Those aspirin probably saved my life, thinning my blood enough to allow it to go through my brain.

The next day had been exhausting and so were the weeks that followed. I mentioned to my mother that I thought I might have had a heart attack, and she thought I should see a doctor.

As I have never been one to run to the doctor, I began practicing a more regular bedtime, drinking more water, taking vitamins, and exercising. Thinking I was just run down, I decided to give my body a rest. And besides, we had no health insurance.

So the symptoms had been all around me. Funny how we don't take notice sometimes until it's too late. Now I try to notice everything—the little things—and I am grateful for them, like children playing and laughing on my backyard swing; the wonderful smell of pizza baking in my old gas range; ice cold lemonade on a hot, sultry day; a phone call from an old friend; the smell of paint on my brushes when the sun is just peeking into my studio; the ability to walk across the room without help; the ability to drive my little car . . . everything. What a wondrous world we've been given!

Forgiveness. It's a funny thing, yet a serious thing. My son, Michael, his wife, Kelly, and my little two-year-old grandson, Jarod, flew in for a visit. There had always been this nagging unforgiveness between my daughter-in-law, Kelly, and me, but now here she was with me—every day for ten days. When the time came for them to return to Ohio and their jobs, I didn't know when or if I would see them again.

Before they left, I called Kelly to my bedside. I told her, "Whatever was between us is over. I can see that you are a wonderful wife and mother, and I'm sorry." She blinked and said, "That's it?" I said, "That's it" to which she replied, "That was easy!" I smiled at her and felt genuine love and warmth. And to this day and forever, our past has remained in the past.

If you have unforgiveness in your heart, get rid of it. It will destroy you and rob you of loving relationships. Life is so very, very precious. I have come to realize that faith, family, and friends are all that matters in this lifetime; nothing else goes with us—not cars, diamonds, money, properties… just love. And *we* are God's instruments of love.

It was a Thursday evening, ten days since the operation, and back they sent me to another hospital for rehabilitation. I was starting to know those ambulance drivers pretty well. The back of the transport vehicle was very hot, and the gurney became soaked with my sweat—but it wasn't only because it was hot inside the vehicle; a fever was also beginning to rage inside my body.

Rehabilitation was set to begin the next day, but I couldn't see how that was going to work out when simply standing made me sick. My head would pound, my blood pressure would drop "off the scale," and I would pass out anytime they stood me up.

My sisters, Bonnie and Peggy, were with me. (I am blessed with wonderful siblings who are not just family but true friends.) While friends and family came to visit, my daughter stayed right by my side. My mother and father called. I didn't want them to see me like this. I held to the belief that I would need them more "when I get home."

A precious nurse named Maria would bathe me at midnight. She would pull out photos of her children from her pockets and tell me all about them. I always felt better after Maria had been there. All of the nursing staff was phenomenal.

For some reason, I kept running fevers. It was hard to eat, and even though the hospital prepared nutritious and pretty tasty food, only some crackers during the night sounded good whenever the fevers would tend to slow.

An internal doctor came to see me. She was concerned about the fevers. She did a spinal tap and put me on some pretty strong antibiotics. After a few days of this, my veins began to collapse. That's when they put in a PIC line that ran directly into my heart. A male nurse named Alan worked on me, and he was ever so gentle.

But despite the tender care I received from the doctors and nurses, I was not getting better. Now I could no longer sit up in bed. It was difficult even for me to move in bed, so the nurses had to move me. The fevers would come and go, but mostly stay. A second spinal tap revealed meningitis.

I seemed to be just barely hanging on. I so wanted to sketch. I wanted to move, but there was no strength, and my head felt like there was rocks in it. Light and sound were extremely painful. The new PIC line collapsed, and they had to put in another one.

My daughter was there the entire time. Thank God for her sweet face. I was so thankful to know the hallucinations in the recovery room had been just that.

On Mother's Day, my daughter brought in her two little girls to visit. Hannah, who is four and a clone of me, and Gracie, who is two, beautiful yet extremely ornery, were unusually quiet. I'm certain Christie must have given them "orders." Hannah sat by my bed, stroking my arm. I peered at her through the bars of my bed. I held onto the rail as she gently put her tiny hand on mine. "I love you so much, Mimi," she said. And then in her typical four-year-old voice, "Ooh, you have tape balls. Can I pick them off?" I had to laugh, as she picked at them one by one.

Days passed without my being able to move. I continued to get sicker and sicker. My head and body were racked with pain. Fevers still raged within me. It was time for another MRI. My daughter walked beside the gurney, but they wouldn't let her in the room. She

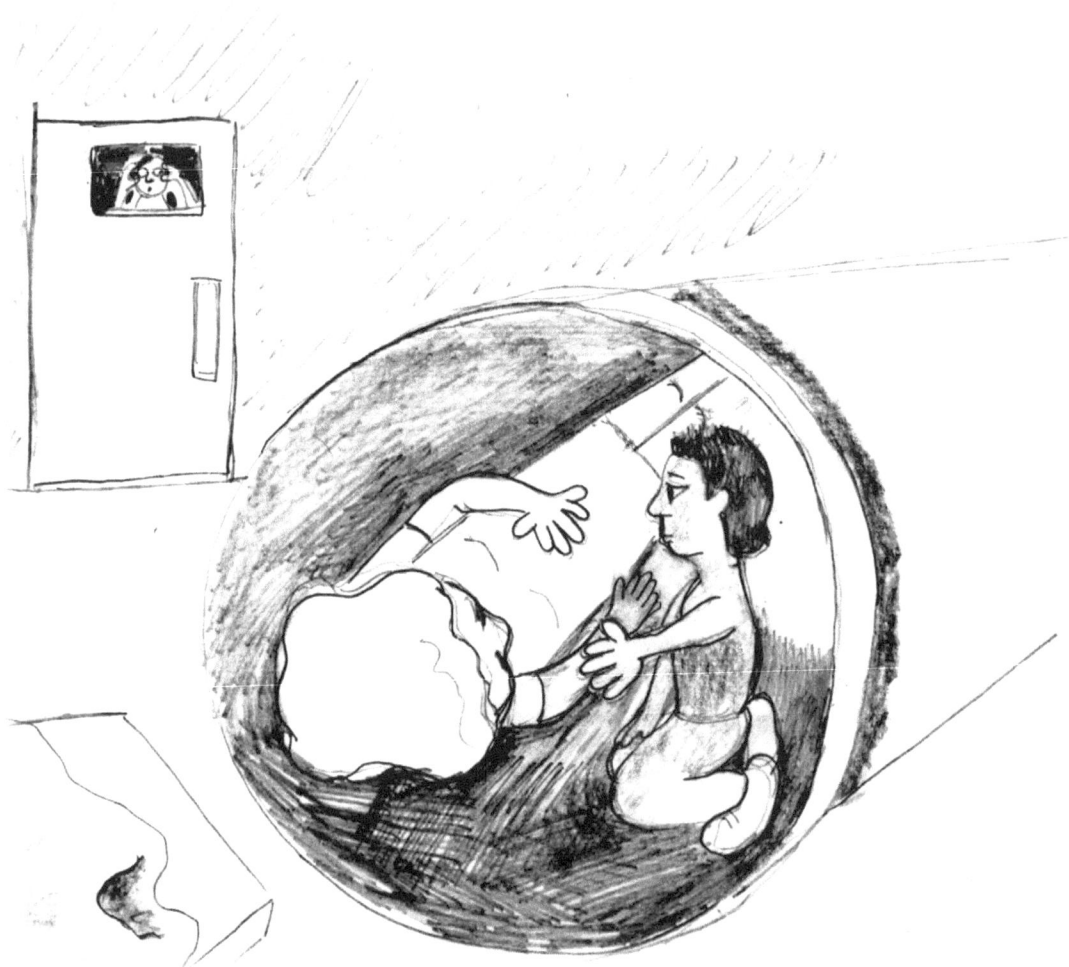

My son, Scottie, "with me" in the MRI tunnel

peered through the window. I had my grandchildren's bunnies with me. They had been with me since Easter.

The technicians were explaining the MRI procedures to me as they were putting me "in the tunnel," but I heard none of it, as I could hardly stand the pain. I felt like I was dying. I started to convulse.

And then—ever so quietly—there was my Scottie, kneeling in the tunnel with me. He appeared to be about twenty-one years old, just like in the photo I have of him on his twenty-first birthday where he's blowing out the candles on his cake. I thought to myself, *He has the most beautiful smile*. He began by saying, "Mom, I've come to take you home," to which I replied, "It's not my time yet, Scottie. I have too much to do." "Mom," he explained, "It's not your call." He began quoting the 23rd Psalm, and when he came to the verse, "Yea though I walk through the valley of the shadow of death, I will fear no evil, for Thou art with me," my spirit was calm even though I knew I was dying. Medical reports reveal that at that exact time, my organs shut down, my left lung collapsed, and I "coded blue." I was on my way to eternity!

Scottie bent down towards my face and kissed my cheek. Scottie's face was whiter than any white I had ever seen. It was if I were to put my hands on his cheek, my hand would disappear into the light.

"No, no, I have too many paintings to paint!" my mind was screaming as we traveled slowly towards the light beyond Scottie's right shoulder. And then—ever so slowly—we traveled back, and once again I was in "the tunnel."

It was at that moment when Christie cried out with a piercing scream outside the door for the nurses to get me out of there.

Later, people asked me about that experience. They wanted to know if I had left my body. I didn't think I had. But when I was asked to sketch what I saw and felt, lo and behold, the sketch revealed that I truly had been hovering over my body! There it was "in black and white."

Here is something you need to know about God. He will walk on water to get to you. He will pass through walls. When His child needs Him, He will do whatever it takes. As parents we've all stood back and watched our toddlers fall when learning to walk, but if that child lets out a cry or gets a bump, with one big swoop we pick him up, pat him, comfort him, and have him try again, right? Well, that's how God was throughout my Jonah experience. He gently nudged me, then watched and waited, but He never took His protective eye off of me.

It was Mother's Day again, and my surgeon, Dr. Foote, had arrived for the first time at my restaurant to enjoy dinner with his mother. Kelly Foote, M.D., is a kind and gentle doctor, one who cares deeply for his patients. As he walked in, he leaned across the podium and asked my husband how I was doing. Jimmy told him that I wasn't doing too well. (I am told that by this time, I had been in the fetal position for several days and was slipping further away with each hour that passed. Attempts to contact the hospital's neurosurgeon had been unsuccessful, but the nursing staff was trying the best they could to get me better, or at least to stabilize me.) Dr. Foote made a phone call, and within minutes I was readied for transport and enroute to his hospital. These ambulance drivers were starting to feel like family.

I was admitted to "the pod," the critical, intensive area of the hospital—only one doctor per patient, 'round the clock. They gave me injections in my stomach—injections of insulin, steroids, all the things my body was supposed to be producing on its own but was not. My left side felt like it was on fire. I learned that my lung had collapsed.

It could have been the new medicines, perhaps the infection was leaving my body, or maybe it was simply God's healing hand, but while in "the pod," I started to feel better. A nurse washed my long hair with dry shampoo. My hair felt gummy from the fevers. Jonah's hair probably got pretty gummy, too. Can you imagine the acid in a whale's belly? Or perhaps God had him in a dry place. Either way, Jonah's experience led him to God, just like mine did.

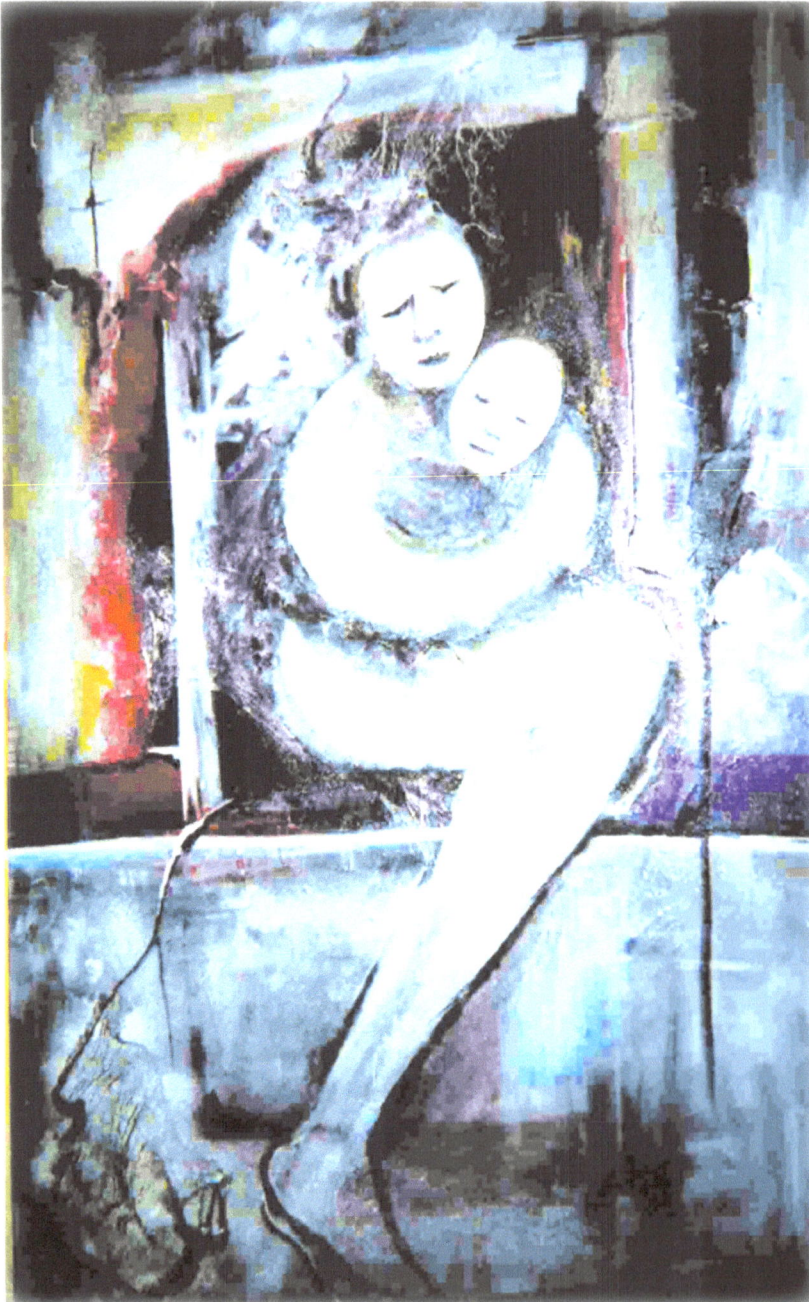

"Shroud of Innocence," a Linda M. Brandt original

After five days of getting healthier, I was ready to start getting stronger. Once again I was transported back to the first hospital for rehabilitation. This was a lifestyle, a whole new world that I never knew existed—one where patients routinely traveled back and forth between hospitals. And there were so many kind people in this world. The driver even stopped at a Wendy's and got me a Coke with lots of ice. It tasted really good. (Who would ever have guessed I'd be going through the drive-through in the back of a medical transport vehicle?) I was on the gurney when the driver handed me his card and told me that after I get out of the hospital, if I ever need anything to just give him a call.

We arrived back at the first hospital after about two hours. What happened next was something the driver said he had never seen before. Six nurses who had helped me initially during rehab and during my bout with spinal meningitis came running out. They took the gurney out of the back of the transport vehicle with me on it and told me excitedly how they had my "suite" all ready for me. They had taken care of my plants and my stuffed animals and were so glad to see me that they hugged and kissed me! These nurses were the most wonderful caregivers.

Then began the healing process—the grueling work. I'm told for every week a person is down and in bed, it takes four weeks to get "back." The first few days of therapy began in the wheelchair, then a belt around my waist, then finally on my feet with a nurse at each side. They played games with me and tried to help me walk. The room wouldn't stop spinning, and my body trembled. I sketched when I could. I wanted my drawings to reveal my transformation. I could hardly hold a pencil, but I had to draw. I had to put my thoughts to paper. Struggling and shaky but determined, I held the little book brought to me by one of my art students.

Seven weeks in critical care. What did my spirit experience? I sketched. I erased. My hand just didn't want to cooperate, but I continued. Seven thumbnails of my experience. I titled them, "7 Weeks: Tragedy to Triumph." My head felt like Jell-o$^{®}$ with big, bumpy rocks inside! I dubbed myself Linda Lump, whose head is like a box of rocks!

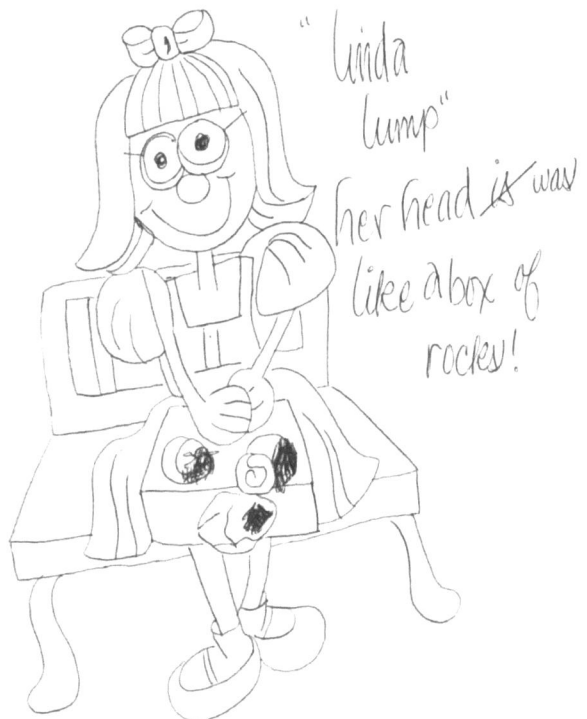

"Linda Lump"

"7 Weeks....Tragedy to Triumph"
and 4 Years

© 2011
Created 2007-2011

7 36" x 48" handmade paints on canvas
by Artist Linda M. Brandt

1. "Le destin a tape' fort".......("Side-Blinded")
2. "il faut tenir le coup".......(" Hanging On")
3. "Elle a entendu"........("She Heard")
4. "La survivante"...... ("Survivor")
5. "Les premières lueurs de l'aube"...("Dawning 1")
6. "Évolution".....("Evolution")
7. "Bien-portante".....("Wellness")

THUMBNAILS

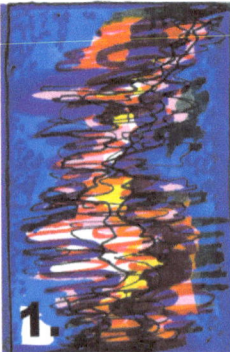

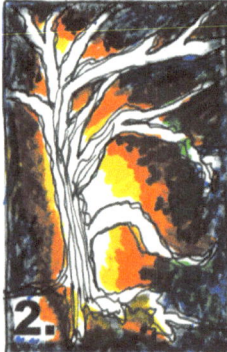

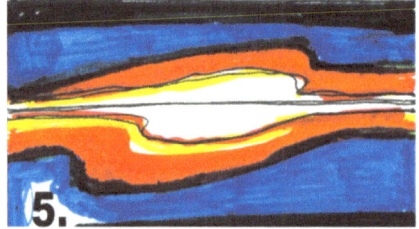

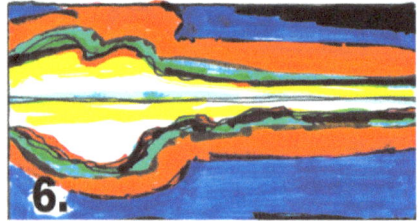

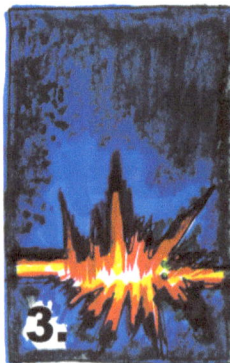

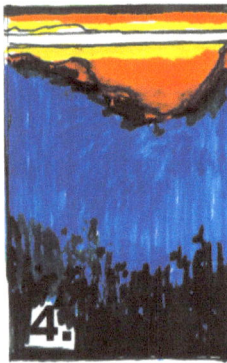

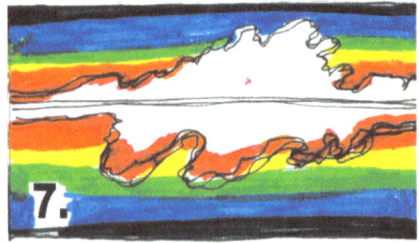

*Please note that because of a very serious brain tumor and it's removal, this work has taken me nearly four years to produce. (nearly 25% of my brain was removed in the process). Six in the collection are in the completion stage and, as shown, "Survivor" is finished. All seven titles have been translated into French in honor of the chief neurosurgeon's care. -Linda M. Brandt

They gave me putty to try and work with in hopes of regaining strength in my hands. They also put x-tape spots in my room in front of my chair so that I would move my feet onto them. The following week of therapy included a walker for short distances. My body shook with weakness, but my mind was becoming clearer. My friends stopped by. A nurse took me outside and helped me to step up on the curb. I never knew walking could be so difficult, even with the use of a walker.

After ten days, I was dismissed from the hospital. That Friday night, three of my friends carried me up the steps of an art gallery where my work was on display. (They teased the other patrons who were entering that they might want to stay away from the punch. I'm glad they were having such fun!) It was weird to be looking at my newly finished work hanging there in the gallery. Why, it was just four months ago that I had been working on these pieces. Would I ever be able to paint like that again?

My sister and parents came and stayed with me. They left six weeks later, and I stood on the porch and cried as their old, red van pulled out of the drive. What would I do now? I was not the same independent person I had always been. My hair was falling out by the handsful, my face was swollen from steroids, and walking was so very difficult. I couldn't even drive. Paintings had to be created with my left hand. In all my years of painting, I had never even thought of putting a brush in my left hand, yet my paintings were beginning to form legibly with my left side. How ironic it was to me that by my fourth painting, one could not even distinguish it from ones I'd painted years before. I keep those four paintings on my drawing board as a reminder of how far I've come.

The pictures on these two pages are the four watercolor paintings I did when I was learning to paint left-handed.

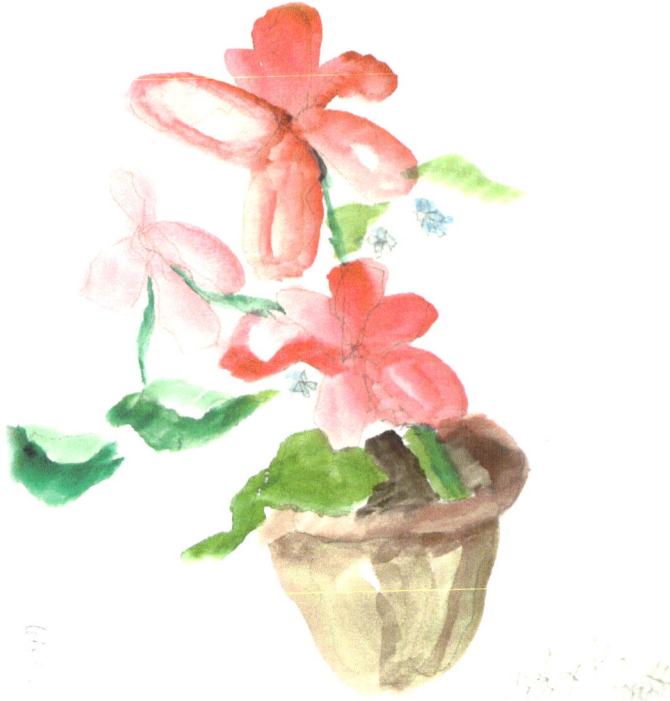

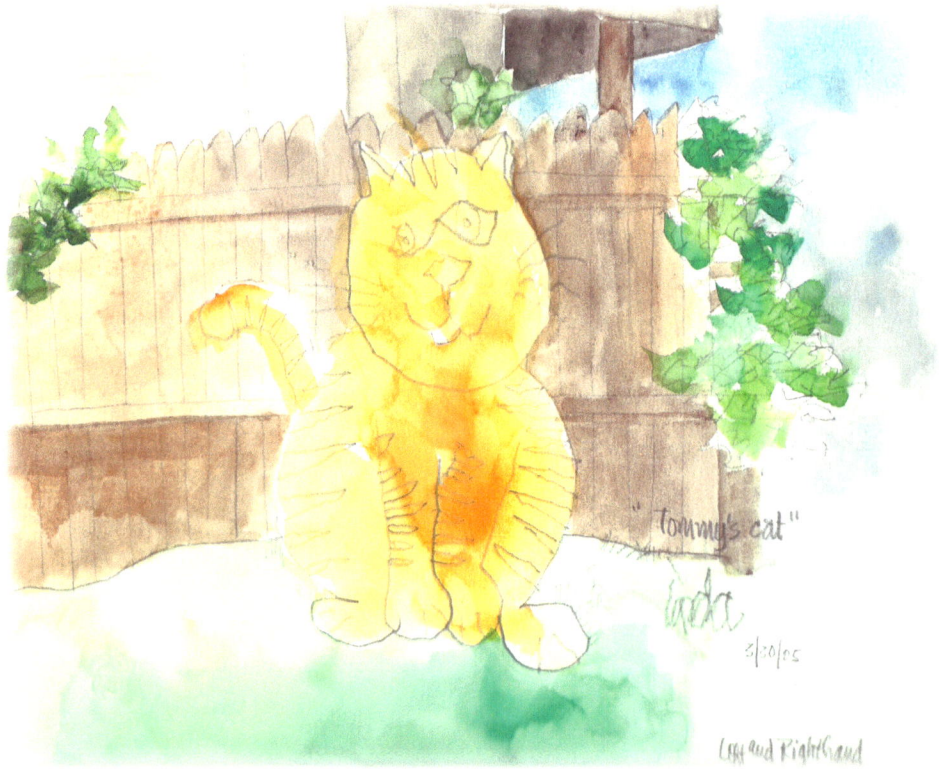

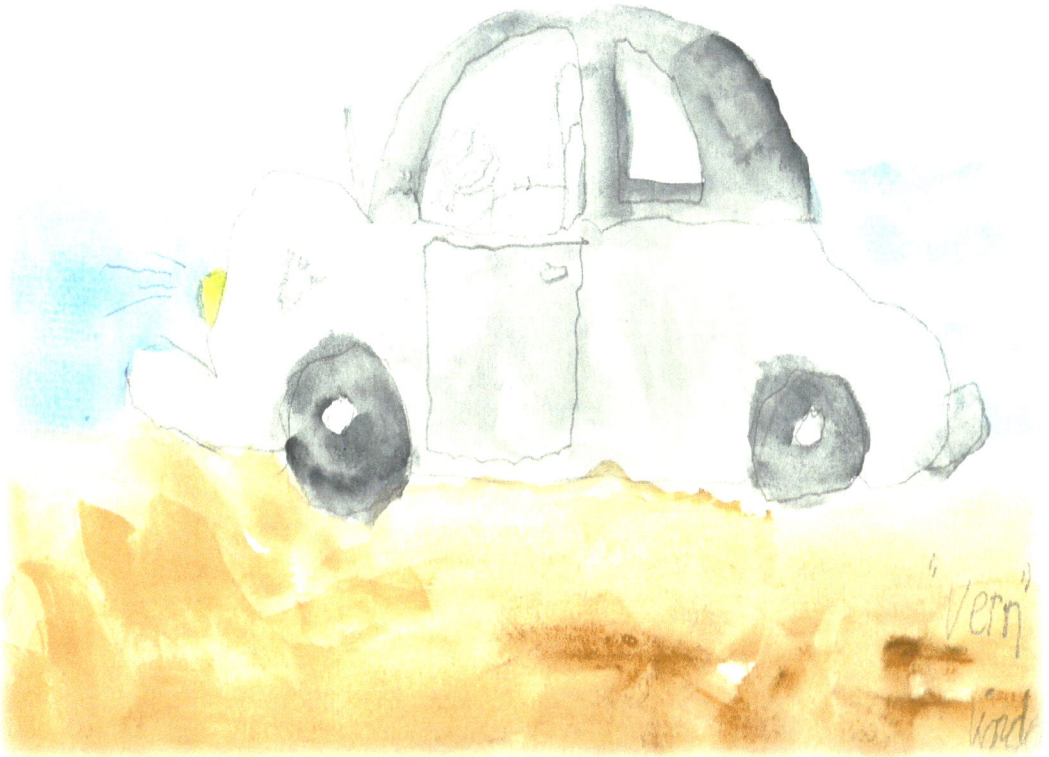

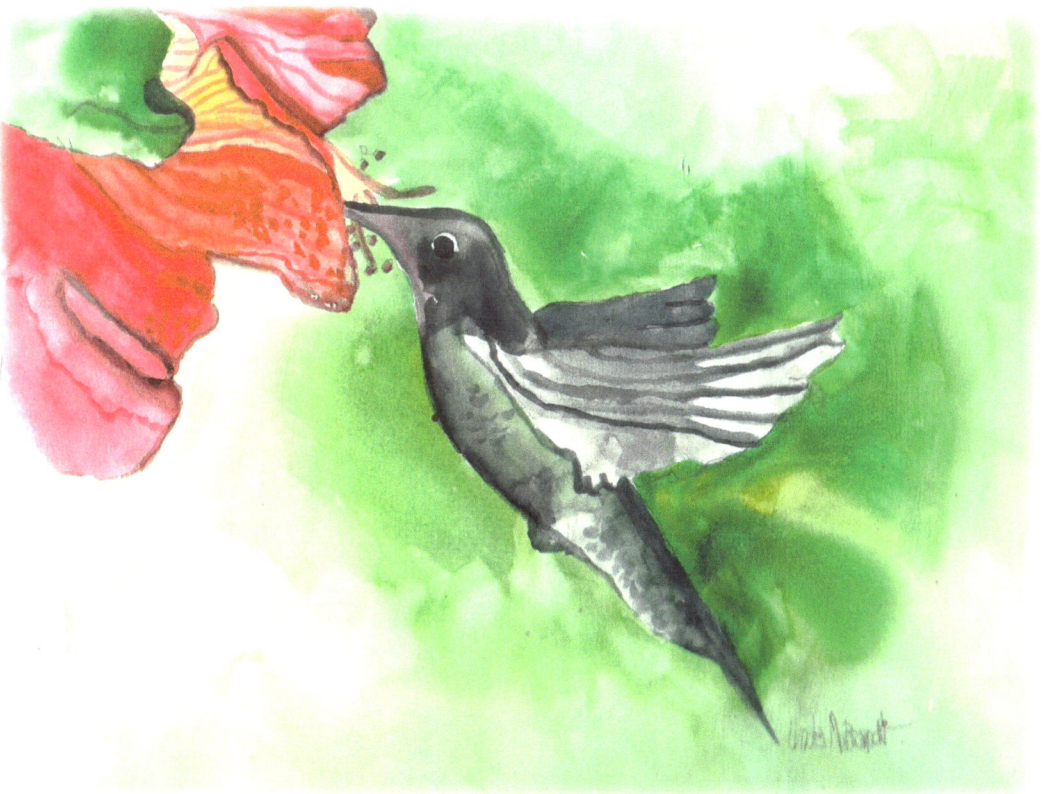

I stood in my studio bewildered. Stacks of canvases—some painted, some bare. Who had painted these, and was it another person who now stood here? Weeks and months went by, and when I sat in front of my makeup mirror, I didn't recognize the person who stared back at me. I hated that new person; I wanted the old Linda back. I still dreamed of dancing and walking in heels.

When I told my friend Greta about my feelings, she gave me some very sage advice. She humbly but sternly reminded me that regardless of how I felt, the old Linda was gone, that this new Linda was a very precious soul, and if I could just learn to love her, my life would change. When she left that morning, I climbed back onto my makeup chair. There, looking back at me in the mirror, was a swollen-faced, shaky, balding woman. I began with, "I still don't know who you are, and I'm not sure I like you, but I guess I'm stuck with you, so I've decided to love you regardless." In that instant, I felt an enormous weight lifted off of me. I would be okay. God would not let me down. An unexplainable peace flooded my soul.

Family would not give up on me. My sisters, Bonnie and Barbie, came down to stay with me and take care of me. They scooped me up, read to me, walked with me (I with a walker), cooked nutritional meals for me, and loved and prayed for me. In the months that followed, I began driving with my friend Annie. I learned to paint again using only my left hand. There were beach walks with friends and lots of card games, dice games, movies, and home-cooked foods. Greta came to do yoga and Pilates with me every day. (She would let me stop to rest for a few minutes, but she would never let me "stop.") There was lots of sweeping as my therapy. Left-to-right action helped to rewire my brain. Cranial massage, acupuncture, herbs, and vitamins were all part of my daily therapy. The first time I baked a cake again, my mother called. When she asked me what I was doing, I told her I was baking a cake, and with that I said, "Oh the cake!" I immediately took it out of the oven and turned it upside down on the cooling rack. Turns out, it had only been in the oven for ten minutes, so cake batter ran down the cabinet and onto the floor. I figured I had better wait for a while to tackle baking.

AFTERWORD

Today I walk without help, mostly without a cane, and only with a slight limp. When I'm tired, walking is more difficult. Some days, even brushing my teeth is tiring! I still need to rest in the afternoons, and sometimes in the mornings, too. In addition to painting, I also speak before audiences and even write and illustrate books for myself and others.

In 2006, a little TV production I wrote thirteen years earlier, *Henry's Life as a Tulip Bulb: Developing an Attitude of Gratitude* became a book. Fully illustrated in my pen & ink and watercolors, it has become the first of eight books in a series to be published by Christian publisher, Innovo Publishing. A full-length movie documenting my "Tragedy to Triumph" is currently being produced and will feature animation of Henry the Tulip Bulb.

It took nearly four years to complete a body of paintings entitled, "7 Weeks: Tragedy to Triumph." The installation of paintings was unveiled at a Haven Hospice facility in St. Augustine in the fall of 2012. Sketched while still in hospital critical care, each very large canvas depicts the emotion of my soul and spirit while reeling from death and despair to eventual hope and healing.

In September 2009, I met a wonderful man, Scott Allen Pilny, and I knew immediately that Someone bigger than I was behind it! God brought another Scott Allen into my life, and we were married six months later. This Scott is not a replacement for my son, but he is, I feel, a wink from God that my son is just fine, and now He's giving me another Scott to watch over me while on earth. God's gifts are so very perfect.

I am truly blessed. Doctors tell me I'm credited in medical journals as being the world's only adult survivor of the particular kind of brain tumor I had. Doctors used to say, "People like you—we never see again; they just go into their homes and go away. We are witnessing a miracle." **It was 2004 when I began "my Jonah journey," and I still remember every day to be thankful. God's grace and abundance surround me.** Nothing I have ever done or could ever do would cause me to deserve this measure of goodness.

I can't say that I understand fully all the reasons for the death of my son, Scottie. But I do know this—that even though his physical body died, his spirit lives on and was able to minister to mine in my moment of greatest need. We won't always be able to see the whys and wherefores in the here and now, but one day when we reflect on our lives, we will see a beautifully woven pattern. We will understand and know there was an infinite, intelligent plan for our good and for God's glory. Hallelujah!

Then Jonah prayed to the LORD his God from the fish's belly. [2] And he said:

"I cried out to the LORD because of my affliction,
And He answered me.

"Out of the belly of Sheol I cried,
And You heard my voice.
[3] For You cast me into the deep,
Into the heart of the seas,
And the floods surrounded me;
All Your billows and Your waves passed over me.
[4] Then I said, 'I have been cast out of Your sight;
Yet I will look again toward Your holy temple.'
[5] The waters surrounded me, even to my soul;
The deep closed around me;
Weeds were wrapped around my head.
[6] I went down to the moorings of the mountains;
The earth with its bars closed behind me forever;
Yet You have brought up my life from the pit,
O LORD, my God.

[7] "When my soul fainted within me,
I remembered the LORD;
And my prayer went up to You,
Into Your holy temple.

[8] "Those who regard worthless idols
Forsake their own Mercy.
[9] But I will sacrifice to You
With the voice of thanksgiving;
I will pay what I have vowed.
Salvation is of the LORD." (Jonah 2:1-9)

The following pictures, "Glad Magnolia" and "Happy Hibiscus," were painted since my brain surgery and are a testament to the remarkable way in which God restored my ability to paint. These pieces are in private collections.

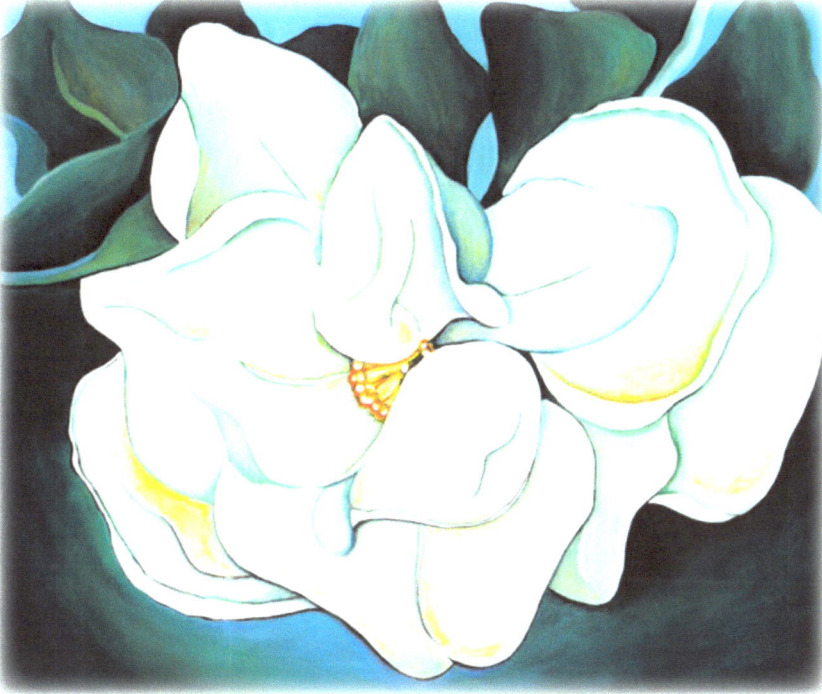

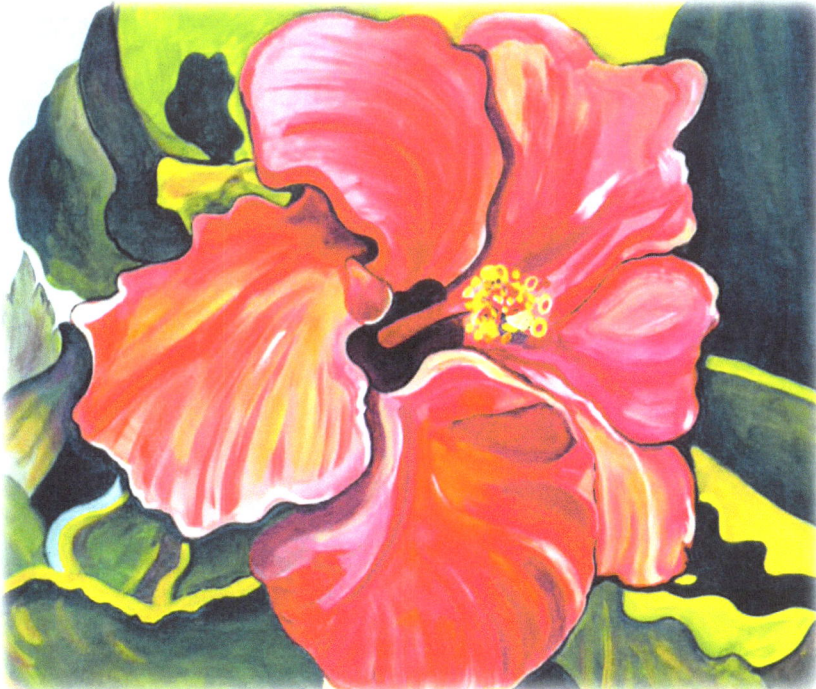

The three paintings shown here hung in The Louvre Museum in Paris, France, as part of a show by The Glendale Gallery.

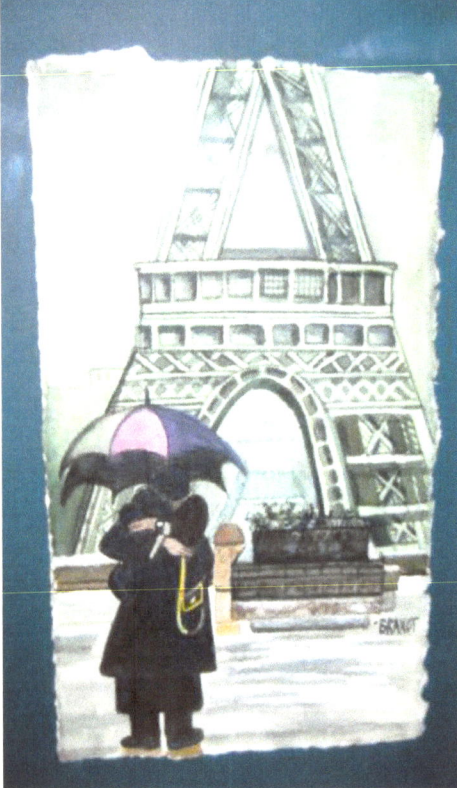

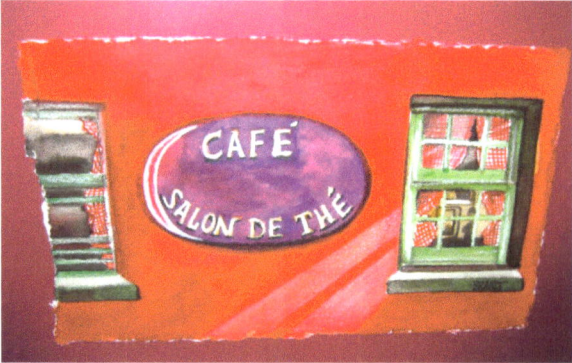

"Endless Time for Lovers"

"Café Salon de Thé"

"Misty Morning at the
        Arc de Triomphe"

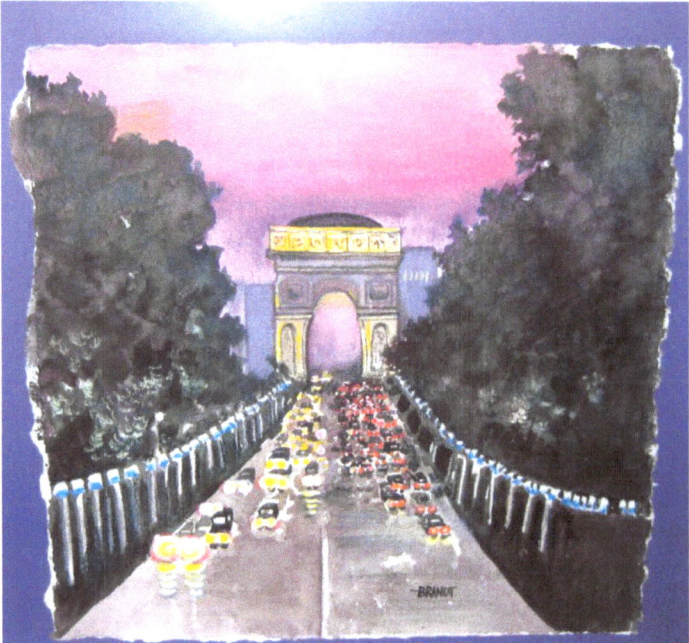

The paintings on the following pages are some of my "fan favorites."

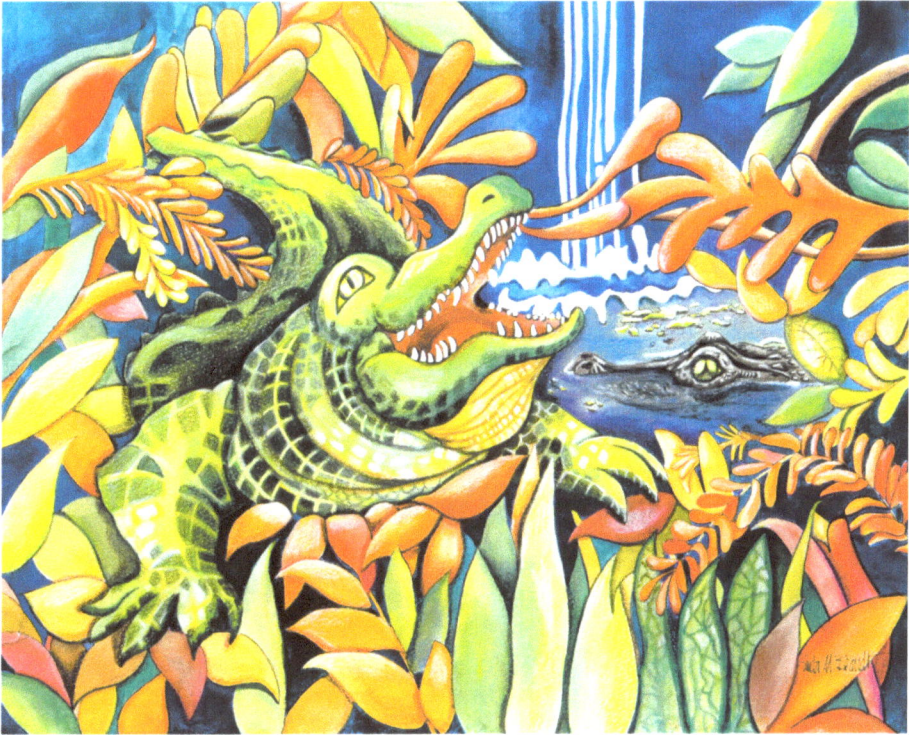

"Gator Time" was purchased by a private individual who gave it to Urban Meyer while he was still head coach of the [University of] Florida Gators.

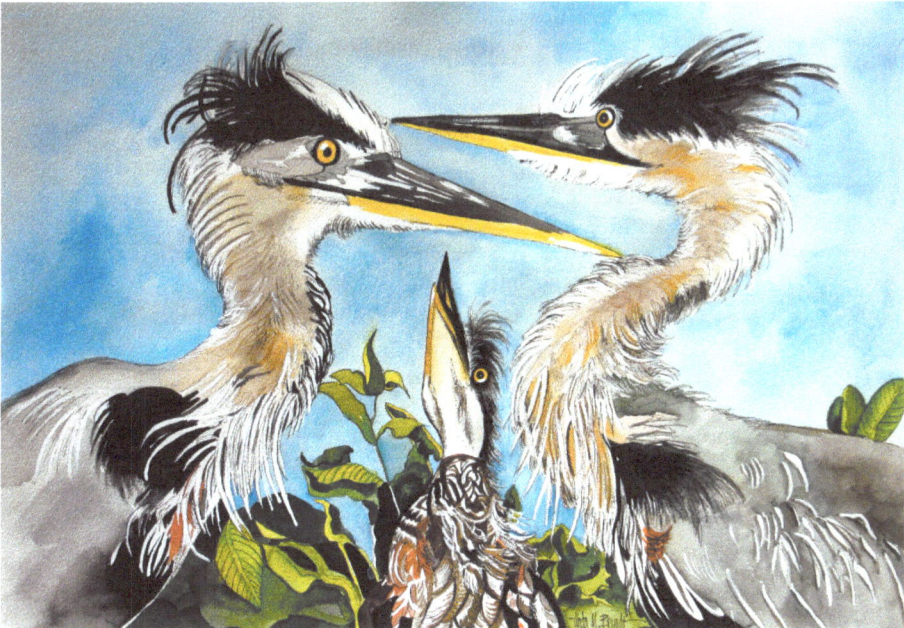

"Larry, Mary, and Mo Tif"

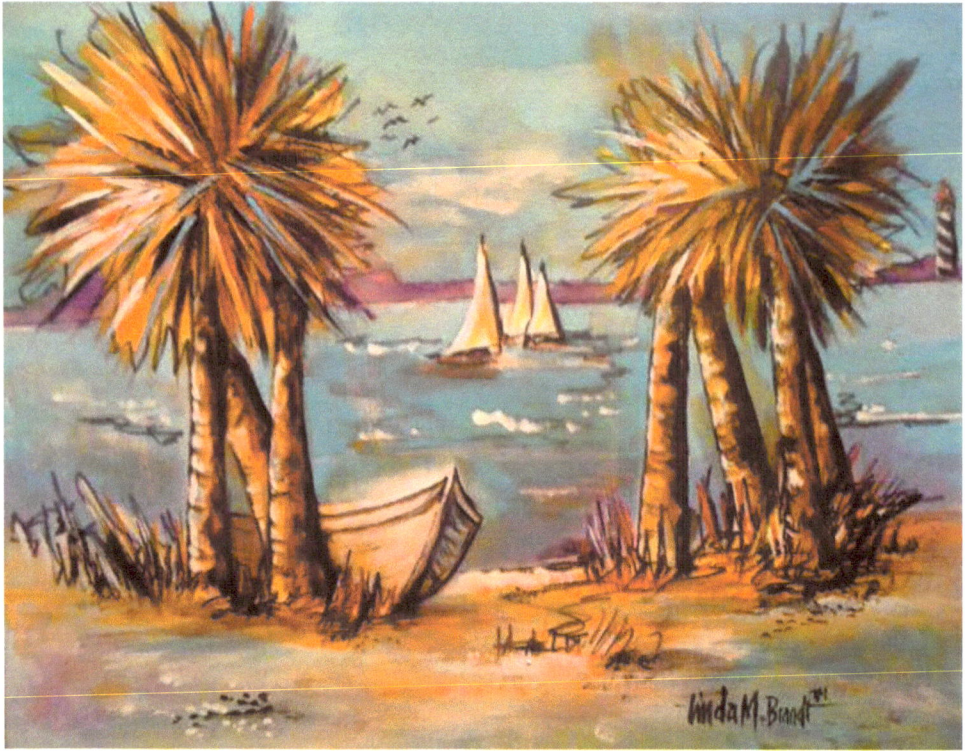

"Saint Augustine Bayfront"

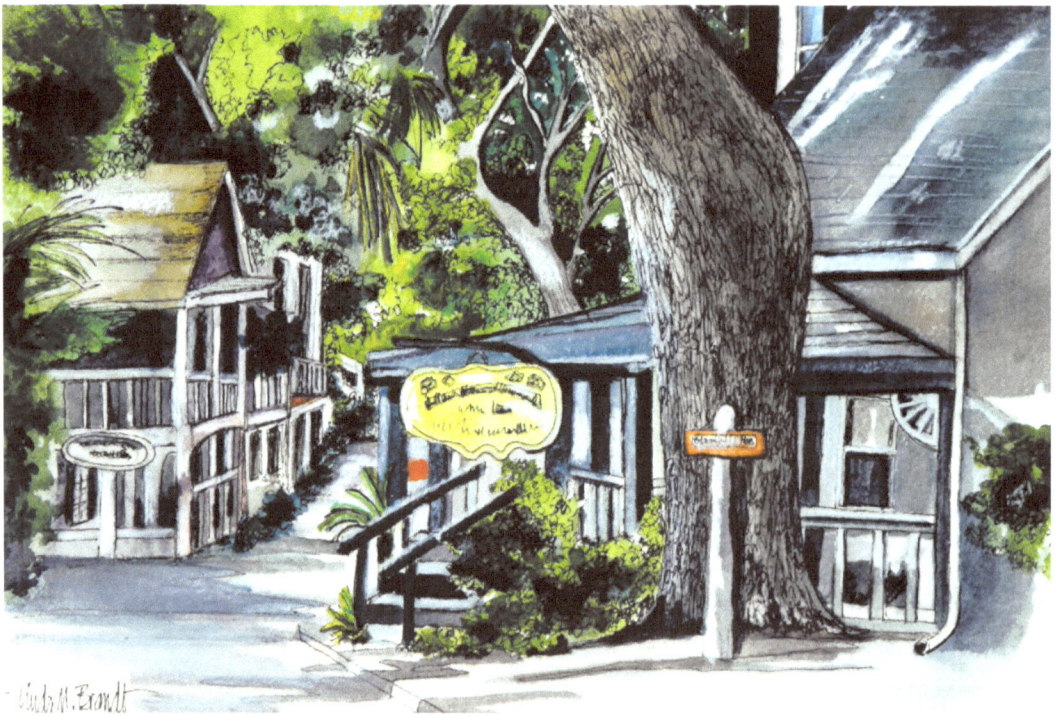

"Side Street in Saint Augustine"

ABOUT THE AUTHOR-ILLUSTRATOR

Having drawn since the age of four, author-artist **Linda M. Brandt** landed her first professional job illustrating political cartoons at the age of nineteen. Her work has been displayed in prestigious venues such as The Louvre, Radio City (NY), Christ Episcopal Church, Haven Hospice, and various U.S. galleries. Many of her paintings are held in private collections around the world including the home of late President Ronald Reagan and past Ohio governor, George Voinovich. Linda is the only known adult survivor of a particular rare and serious brain tumor. Following surgery to remove the tumor, she contracted spinal meningitis and spent two months in hospital critical care. It was during this time, while inside an MRI chamber, that Linda had a near-death experience. With God's help and with the prayers and love of her family and friends, Linda spent the next three years learning to walk again, to drive again, and at last, to paint again. Collectors of her paintings believe her work is even more inspirational and dramatic than before as she emphasizes triumph over tragedy through her art. Linda's speaking engagements relate her experiences of being grateful and how gratitude can affect a person's well-being, both now and in the hereafter.

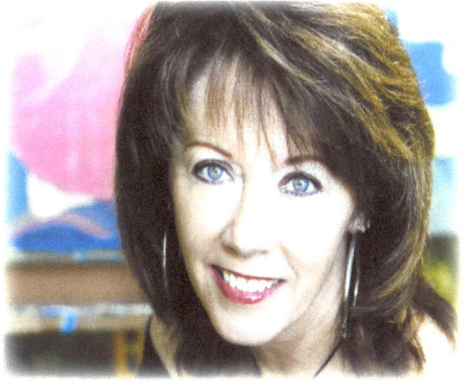

To schedule Linda for book signings, public speaking engagements, or art exhibits, contact info@innovopublishing.com.
1-888-546-2111

Develop in Your Little Ones an
ATTITUDE OF GRATITUDE

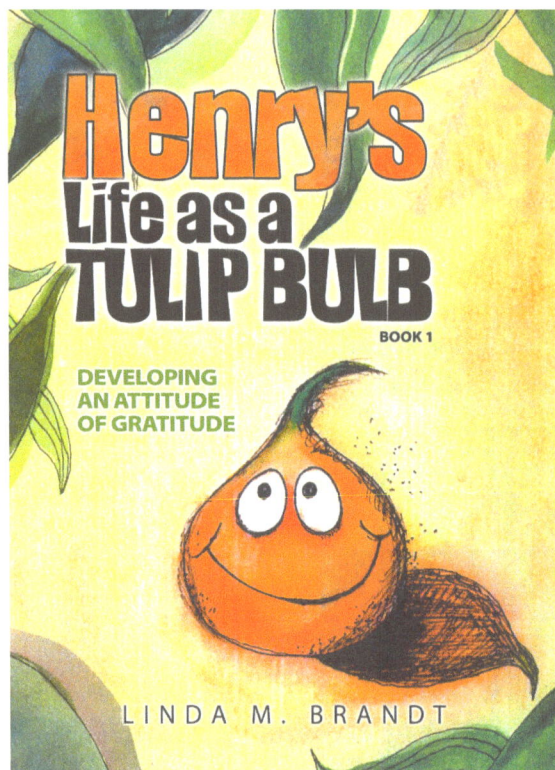

Henry the Tulip Bulb was quite content with his comfortable, happy life on a grocery store shelf, so how would he handle all the changes about to take place when two little girls bought him and took him home to plant him in the cold, cold ground?

Written and illustrated by Linda M. Brandt, *Henry's Life as a Tulip Bulb* is meant to be enjoyed by children of all ages but is an especially excellent read for preschool and early childhood. In his unique and charming way, Henry very cleverly shows how to go beyond merely overcoming adversity to actually developing an attitude of gratitude for those hard times in life that tend to challenge us, break us, and ultimately grow us.

If you marveled at Linda's remarkable life story as recorded in her book, *My Jonah Journey,* then you will certainly want to share *Henry's Life as a Tulib Bulb* with the little ones you love.

Available in hardback, paperback, and eBook editions at www.innovopublishing.com.

More Inspirational Titles from Innovo Publishing

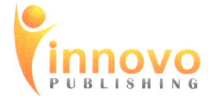

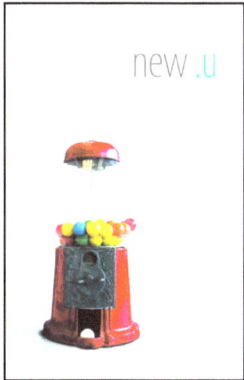

NEW.U by Jason Creech. Are you just getting started as a new Christian? Then you probably have a lot of questions. In this five-week devotional you'll discover a boatload of answers. Learn the simplicity of the Christian life. Welcome to freedom. Welcome to the new you.

ISBN 978-1-936076-64-2 , Paperback, $9.95
Available in eBook editions.

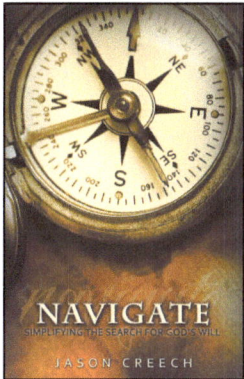

NAVIGATE by Jason Creech. For most of my Christian journey, I've searched for God's will. During the quest, I've faced confusion, anxiety, disappointment, and more trouble than I could ever have anticipated. But maybe I've had it all wrong. Maybe I don't have to search for God's will. Maybe God's will searches for me. Let's explore this idea together. Join me and over two dozen other pilgrims as we simplify the search for God's will. —Jason

ISBN 978-1-936076-67-3, Paperback, $9.95
Available in eBook editions.

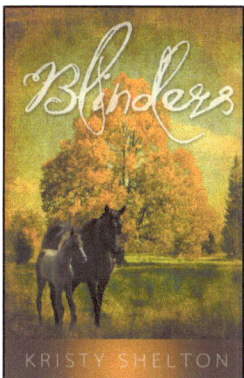

BLINDERS, a novel by Kristy Shelton, portrays a beautiful relationship between a former slave couple, their love for a boy who wanders onto their farm, and the redeeming forgiveness of the heavenly Father.

ISBN 978-1-936076-65-9, Paperback, $12.95
ISBN 978-1-936076-74-1, Hardback, $19.95
Available in eBook editions.

ABOUT INNOVO PUBLISHING LLC

Innovo Publishing LLC is a full-service Christian publishing company serving the Christian and wholesome markets. Innovo creates, distributes, and markets quality books, eBooks, audiobooks, music, and film through traditional and innovative publishing models and services. Innovo provides distribution, marketing, and automated order fulfillment through a network of thousands of physical and online wholesalers, retailers, bookstores, music stores, schools, and libraries worldwide. Innovo provides a unique combination of traditional publishing, co-publishing, and independent (self) publishing arrangements that allow authors, artists, and organizations to accomplish their personal, organizational, and philanthropic publishing goals. Visit Innovo Publishing's web site at www.innovopublishing. com or email Innovo at info@innovopublishing.com.

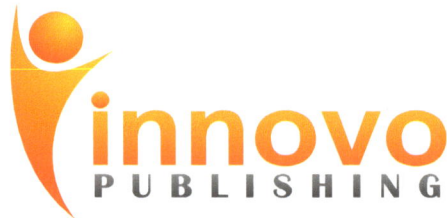

www.ingramcontent.com/pod-product-compliance
Lightning Source LLC
Chambersburg PA
CBHW060819270326
41930CB00002B/90